Pegan Diet Smoothies

100% VEGAN

Delicious Plant-Based Paleo Smoothie Recipes for Vibrant Health, Abundant Energy, and Natural Weight Loss

Copyright ©Karen Greenvang 2019

All rights reserved. No part of this publication may be reproduced, stored in a retrieval system, or transmitted, in any form or by any means, electronic, mechanical, photocopying, recording or otherwise, without the prior written permission of the author and the publishers.

The scanning, uploading, and distribution of this book via the Internet, or via any other means, without the permission of the author is illegal and punishable by law. Please purchase only authorized electronic editions, and do not participate in or encourage electronic piracy of copyrighted materials.

All information in this book has been carefully researched and checked for factual accuracy. However, the author and publishers make no warranty, expressed or implied, that the information contained herein is appropriate for every individual, situation or purpose, and assume no responsibility for errors or omission. The reader assumes the risk and full responsibility for all actions, and the author will not be held liable for any loss or damage, whether consequential, incidental, and special or otherwise, that may result from the information presented in this publication.

All cooking is an experiment in a sense, and many people come to the same or similar recipe over time. All recipes in this book have been derived from author's personal experience. Should any bear a close resemblance to those used elsewhere, that is purely coincidental.

The book is not intended to provide medical advice or to take the place of medical advice and treatment from your personal physician. Readers are advised to consult their own doctors or other qualified health professionals regarding the treatment of medical conditions. The author shall not be held liable or responsible for any misunderstanding or misuse of the information contained in this book. The information is not intended to diagnose, treat or cure any disease.

It is important to remember that the author of this book is not a doctor/ medical professional. Only opinions based upon her own personal experiences or research are cited. THE AUTHOR DOES NOT OFFER MEDICAL ADVICE or prescribe any treatments. For any health or medical issues – you should be talking to your doctor first.

Contents

Ready to Transform Your Wellbeing?...................................... 9

Pegan Smoothies- Food List & Shopping List................... 18

    Recipe #1 Tropical Green Coconut Smoothie.............. 25

    Recipe # 2 Detox Berry Smoothie................................ 26

    Recipe #3 Cashew Date Guilt-Free Treat..................... 27

    Recipe #4 High Energy Creamy Protein Smoothie...... 28

    Recipe #5 Apple Cinnamon Aphrodisiac Smoothie..... 29

    Recipe #6 Hydration Refreshment Protein Smoothie 30

    Recipe #7 Easy Sweet Green Smoothie....................... 31

    Recipe #8 Sweet Anti-Inflammatory Smoothie.......... 32

    Recipe #9 Mediterranean Health Alkaline Smoothie. 33

    Recipe #10 Cilantro Detox Smoothie........................... 35

    Recipe #11 Pegan Weight Loss Smoothie.................... 36

    Recipe #12 Keto Pegan Energy Detox Smoothie........ 37

    Recipe #13 Healthy Eyes Keto Pegan Smoothie......... 38

    Recipe#14 Easy Lemon Detox Smoothie..................... 39

Recipe #15 Easy Vegan Paleo Relaxation Smoothie ... 40

Recipe #16 Spice It Up Mediterranean Smoothie 41

Recipe #17 Optimal Balance Smoothie 42

Recipe #18 Almond Protein Smoothie........................ 43

Recipe #19 Creamy Energy Alkaline Pegan Smoothie 44

Recipe #20 Vegan Paleo Liver Lover Smoothie........... 45

Recipe #21 Cilantro Antioxidant Smoothie 46

Recipe #22 Vitamin C Sweetness Smoothie 47

Recipe #23 Superfood Protein Smoothie 48

Recipe #24 Green Coconut Smoothie 50

Recipe #25 Cinnamon Sweetness Smoothie............... 51

Recipe #26 Green Tea Fat Burn Smoothie 52

Recipe #27 Natural Beauty Vegan Paleo Smoothie.... 53

Recipe #28 Spicy Antioxidant Smoothie 54

Recipe #29 Hormone Rebalancer Smoothie 55

Recipe #30 Mineral Dream Smoothie......................... 56

Recipe #31 Creamy Alkaline Spicy Smoothie.............. 57

Recipe #32 Fresh Basil Antioxidant Smoothie 58

Recipe #33 Arugula Protein Smoothie 59

Recipe #34 Carrot Orange Protein Pegan Smoothie ... 60

Recipe #35 Easy Refreshment Smoothie 61

Recipe #36 Green Mediterranean Smoothie 62

Recipe #37 Super Irion Smoothie 63

Recipe #38 Good Fat Good Protein Pegan Smoothie . 64

Recipe #39 Creamy Papaya Refreshment Smoothie .. 65

Recipe #40 Easy Fat Burn Pineapple Smoothie 66

Recipe #41 Natural Detox Soup Style Smoothie 67

Recipe #42 Exotic Soup Style Smoothie 69

Recipe #43 Dried Fruit Dream Smoothie 71

Recipe #44 White Chia Smoothie 72

Recipe #45 Delicious Thai Style Smoothie 73

Recipe #46 Nutritious Vanilla Smoothie 75

Recipe #47 Seduction Cinnamon Smoothie 77

Recipe #48 Ashwagandha Herbal Delight Smoothie .. 78

In Conclusion 80

Special Offer from Karen- VIP Reader Newsletter......... 82

More Books Written by Karen Greenvang 83

Ready to Transform Your Wellbeing?

Thank you so much for taking an interest in this book.

My name is Karen and I write easy-to-follow vegan recipe books to help people live a healthier and more conscious lifestyle.

A couple of years ago I wrote the first book in the Pegan Diet (Vegan Paleo) book series:

Pegan Diet Cookbook: 100% VEGAN: Your Personalized Guide to Losing Weight, Reducing Inflammation, and Feeling Amazing

After talking to my readers and email newsletter subscribers, I realized that many people benefited from delicious and nutritious plant-based paleo recipes I was sharing. At the same time, people really appreciated the pegan smoothie recipes. Hence, I decided to write this book- to share my best pegan diet friendly smoothie recipes to help you create vibrant health.

As all my books in the vegan diet and lifestyle series, Pegan Diet Smoothies is very practical, and easy to follow, even for a total beginner. At the same time, a health veteran will also surely find new ideas, blends and combinations to spice up their smoothie routine.

So what exactly is a pegan diet?

The Pegan diet is where the concepts of vegan and paleo meet. It has many health benefits that will help you sustain a healthy lifestyle based around a nutritionally sound way of eating. The pegan diet consists of mainly fruits, vegetables, nuts, seeds, avocados, olives, and coconut. Grains, legumes and soy products are excluded as they all require some form of processing. Any form of refined sugars is also excluded.

There are many benefits to a pegan diet that include a low glycemic load as refined carbohydrates of any kind are excluded. The high density of fresh fruits and vegetables provide essential vitamins, minerals and fiber. The nuts, seeds, avocados, olives and coconut provide heart healthy, good quality fats. One would think that the pegan diet would be lacking in protein, but you will be getting a sufficient amount of this essential dietary component from the nuts which form a part of most of the recipes.

So, to make it simple, the recipes contained in this book are both vegan-friendly and paleo friendly. They are also naturally gluten-free.

This book is an excellent choice for:

-vegans and vegetarians

-anyone interested in a healthy, whole food, plant-based lifestyle

-anyone wishing to add more fresh fruits and vegetables into their diets

-paleo diet followers who would like to explore more of a gatherer's side of this diet

-gluten-free diet followers

-anyone wishing to restore natural energy via fresh, plant-based foods

The recipes in this book will give you inspiration and an abundance of delicious and nutritious vegan paleo smoothies.

The beauty of pegan recipes is that they create meals that are very easy to have on the go since they consist of such simple and basic ingredients.

If you feel sick and tired of feeling sick and tired and wish to restore energy and zest for life, try to eat a pegan diet for at least a week. At the same time, remember to drink plenty of water and eliminate caffeine and sugar drinks. Even if you eat this way 80% of the time, you will still be able to energize yourself. Personally, I eat a fully vegan diet as this is my personal choice. My vegan diet is balanced, but I like to focus on pegan recipes or raw food recipes whenever I need more energy- I usually go pegan (grain free, no legumes, no process foods and I eat mostly raw or only slightly cooked pegan style recipes) for a week or two, whenever my body needs it. Or, I simply try to add more raw, unprocessed foods into my diet. These are both vegan (no animal products) and paleo-gatherer (no grains, no soy, no legumes, no gluten) friendly.

This is the best of the 2 worlds!

Simplicity Means Health Success!

After surveying my readers, I have quickly identified that most of them were looking for quick and easy recipes. Something "simple to follow". It made so much sense to me.

Smoothies are the best solution, because they can be created quickly and easily, even if a person is not an experienced chef.

The best part? They are even easier to make than salads. And it takes much less time to go through them…

We are talking about tasty, delicious and nutritious pegan smoothies you will never get bored with. Smoothies that are healing and rich in natural protein and good fats while offering a variety of taste, from spicy to sweet.

Whether you are just starting out, or are a vegan veteran looking for new recipes, or perhaps you want to start eating less of processed foods while adding an abundance of healing, nutrient rich recipes- you have come to the right place.

My mistakes with a vegan diet

I'll be honest with you because I am not ashamed of admitting my mistakes. We are in this together and it is my hope that by admitting what I did wrong with my diet you can avoid my early mistakes.

When I first got started on a vegan diet, I ate way too many processed foods. I was happy I stopped eating animal products, however I did not make any effort to learn about balanced vegan nutrition. And I still hated eating veggies.

So, I was living on a vegan junk food, sugar, processed carbs, coffee and soda.

Because of that, I was feeling tired all the time. It was only when I started transitioning to a fresh, plant-based, unprocessed diet, that I was able to create unstoppable energy through a balanced, whole food vegan diet. Pegan diet smoothies was one of the tools I turned to, and am still using.

And it's thanks to that "unstoppable energy" I can use my free time to create healthy vegan plant-based recipe guides like this one.

Every now and then, I still treat myself to vegan junk food. It's absolutely fine as a treat.

But, it feels good to know I have my balanced, vegan, plant-based plan to follow and a foundation that is fresh, clean, vegan diet that helps me revitalize my mind and body. I no longer need to drink coffee to keep me going. I drink it every now and then because I enjoy it. However, I no longer need it to function as a normal human being.

The good news? You can get hooked on healthy eating, fruits, veggies and superfoods. When you start adding pegan smoothies to your diet, your mindset and habits will start shifting. Your body will feel happy because you will be feeding it with vital nutrients it needs to stimulate the healing process and give you the nutrition you deserve to create the new, healthier and more empowered you.

The Alkaline Benefit

By drinking more pegan smoothies, you automatically increase your intake of alkaline foods. Here's the simple definition of the alkaline diet:

Our blood's optimal pH should be 7.35-7.4 which is slightly alkaline. By adding more alkaline foods (fresh fruits and veggies that are naturally rich in vitamins and minerals) we help our body regulate its optimal blood pH.

If we fail to do so and we eat processed foods that are acid-forming, we torture our body with incredible stress. If we constantly eat foods that are acid-forming, we eventually get sick as our body can no longer regulate its pH for us. The pegan diet is naturally alkaline-forming and helps us restore energy by creating balance.

The best alkaline foods include:

-fresh veggies and greens

-low-sugar fruits such as limes, lemons, grapefruits

-nuts and seeds such as almonds (and almond milk)

-good plant-based fats, for example flax seed oil and coconut oil

-Himalayan salt (it's very rich in alkaline minerals such as Magnesium).

-herbs and herbal tea (no caffeine)

Surprise surprise! They are also vegan paleo friendly. Needless to say, we will be using them in our Pegan smoothies.

To make it simple - Just eat more fresh fruits and veggies, it's as simple as that. This rule is compatible with all the diets- vegan, vegetarian, paleo, low carb, high carb, gluten free + many more.

To sum up, the alkaline diet (and keep it simple):

alkaline foods are gluten-free, plant-based and naturally low in sugar. Most alkaline diet experts recommend you make about 70% of your diet rich in alkaline-forming foods.

The pegan diet is an excellent, natural tool to help you enrich you diet with easy-to-digest foods that are rich in vitamins, minerals and fiber, including alkaline foods as well as other plant-based, clean foods to create balance.

One of the easiest ways to incorporate more vegan paleo foods into your diet is through smoothies.

With this guide, you will learn a myriad of recipes that follow the vegan paleo rules and include a variety of smoothies such as:

-green smoothies (perfect to add more green, alkalizing foods and leafy greens into your diet)

-detox smoothies – these focus on low sugar fruit and strictly alkaline foods

-protein smoothies – these are great as a meal replacement and will keep you energized, strong and healthy

-soup smoothies- these are smoothies that can be easily turned into a delicious, healing soup (raw or cooked)

-tasty, colorful fruit smoothies – these are amazing as a natural treat. I see them as a gift from God! Natural sweetness is something I am definitely very grateful for.

-naturally sweet treat smoothies (yummy!)

You will discover naturally sweet smoothies, spicy smoothies and savory smoothies. We will even explore oriental taste while learning about the best superfoods that you can use with your vegan paleo smoothie recipes. Don't worry, these superfoods and herbs are easy to find and inexpensive.

Also, by discovering how easy it is to create a simple nutritious smoothie that can be a great meal replacement, you will soon realize you are spending less money on eating out or take-aways. The only thing you need is a decent blender, intention and passion to thrive!

Now, let's have a look at the shipping lists so that you know exactly what ingredients you should be focusing on on your vegan paleo smoothie journey!

Pegan Smoothies- Food List & Shopping List

Fruit:

- all fresh fruit

Strictly alkaline fruit to add to your smoothies:

- Limes
- Lemons
- Grapefruits
- Avocado (yes, it's a fruit)
- Tomato (yea, it's a fruit)
- Pomegranate

Please note- if you are on a low sugar diet, it is recommended you focus more on alkaline fruits because they are naturally low in sugar. If you suffer from any sugar related health problems, be sure to consult a physician to check which recipes from this book are suitable for you.

Recommended Pegan Greens:

- all fresh greens and leafy greens

Pegan Diet Smoothies Introduction

Pegan Veggies:
- All fresh veggies

Greens are very good for you, and if used correctly, they will taste really nice in your smoothies. Don't worry if you have never made any green smoothies, or are not too sure how they will taste. The recipes contained in this book got you covered.

Other fresh leafy greens as well as:
- Parsley
- Mint
- Chive
- Dill

Pegan Spices & Herbs for Your Smoothies:

The following herbs and spices will make your smoothies taste delicious.

They are also full of anti-inflammatory properties.
- Cinnamon
- Himalaya Salt (very rich in alkaline minerals like Magnesium)
- Curry

- Red Chili Powder
- Cumin
- Nutmeg
- Italian spices
- Oregano
- Rosemary
- Lavender
- Mint
- Chamomile
- Fennel
- Cilantro
- Moringa

The smoothie recipes from this book will give you guidelines as for how to use some of the herbs mentioned above to create specific, therapeutic smoothies, such as anti-insomnia smoothie, relaxation smoothie and more.

Pegan Sweeteners and Supplements (Optional):
- Stevia (very helpful if you want to make a sweet smoothie without using sugar or sugar-containing foods or supplements)
- Green Powders

- Moringa Powder
- Maca Powder
- Ashwagandha Powder

Pegan Approved Fats:
- Olive oil (organic, cold-pressed)
- Avocado oil
- Hemp oil
- Flaxseed oil
- Coconut oil
- Sesame oil

Please note, there is no need to purchase all of them, one, or two is enough; my two favorites are coconut oil and olive oil.

You can also add good fats through nuts, seeds and avocado fruits. So, if you prefer to stick to "as natural as possible", you don't need to add any oils to your smoothies, it's really up to you.

Pegan Approved Nuts and Seeds:
- Almonds
- Cashews
- Brazilian Nuts
- Macadamia Nuts

- Walnut
- Pine
- Pistachio
- Hazelnut
- Sunflower seeds
- Chia seeds

+ other (however it's recommended you stay away from peanuts).

Pegan Friendly Milk & Other Liquids to Use in Smoothies:
- Almond milk
- Coconut milk
- Hazelnut milk
- Coconut water
- Herbal infusions
- Organic Apple Cider Vinegar

If you have any questions about the food lists for pegan smoothies, please email me at:

karenveganbooks@gmail.com

Free Vegan Email Newsletter + Bonus Smoothie Guide for You

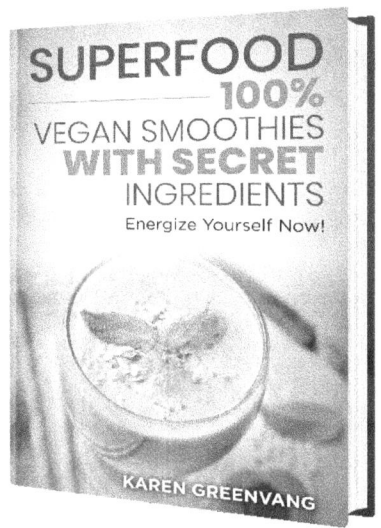

Before we dive into the recipes, I would like to invite you to sign up for my spam free, 100% love-based, vegan email newsletter (I send out fresh vegan recipes, tips and inspiration).

When you sign up, you will receive a free bonus guide with my best vegan superfood smoothie recipes.

Sign up below, it's free:

www.yourwellnessbooks.com/karen-smoothies

(any problems please email me: karenveganbooks@gmail.com)

About the Recipes & the Measurements

The cup measurement I use is the American Cup measurement. I also use it for dry ingredients. If you are new to it, let me help you: If you don't have American Cup measures, just use a metric or imperial liquid measuring jug and fill your jug with your ingredient to the corresponding level. Here's how to go about it:

1 American Cup= 250ml= 8 fl.oz.

For example:
If a recipe calls for 1 cup of almonds, simply place your almonds into your measuring jug until it reaches the 250 ml/8oz mark.
I hope you found it helpful. I know that different countries use different measurements and I wanted to make things simple for you. I have also noticed that very often those who are used to American Cup measurements complain about metric measurements and vice versa. However, if you apply what I have just explained, you will find it easy to use both.

Now, let's dive into the recipes!

Recipe #1 Tropical Green Coconut Smoothie

Both papaya and pineapple are very high in vitamin C, antioxidants and the essential minerals such as potassium, copper and magnesium.

Spinach is highly alkalizing and by blending in nicely with other ingredients, it helps create a beginner friendly, tasty green smoothie.

Almonds and chia seeds add in good protein and fats.

Servings: 2

Ingredients:

- Half cup of fresh papaya, chopped
- Half cup of fresh pineapple, chopped
- A handful of almonds, soaked in water for a few hours
- Half cup of spinach leaves, washed
- 1 cup coconut milk

Instructions:

1. Blend, serve and enjoy!

Recipe # 2 Detox Berry Smoothie

Berries are very high in antioxidants and immune-boosting properties. In this smoothie, they combine their antioxidant benefits with avocados and greens. Avocado adds in good fat and kale is rich in natural protein and chlorophyll. Fresh coconut milk makes this smoothie creamy and delicious.

Servings: 2

Ingredients:

- 1 cup of fresh blueberries
- 1 big avocado, peeled and pitted
- A few slices of lime, peeled
- Half cup of kales leaves, chopped
- 1 cup of chilled coconut milk
- 1 teaspoon cinnamon powder (to garnish)

Instructions:

1.Blend all the ingredients.

2.Serve your smoothie in a big smoothie glass, sprinkle over some cinnamon powder and enjoy!

Recipe #3 Cashew Date Guilt-Free Treat

Are you looking for natural sweetness? Craving something creamy? Try this smoothie! Dates are a great source of the essential minerals iron, calcium, magnesium, zinc; and are very high in fiber. Grapefruits are rich in vitamin C and very alkalizing for the body. This smoothie creates the perfect balance of taste and benefit!

Servings: 2

Ingredients:

- ¼ cup dates, pitted roughly chopped
- 1 grapefruit, peeled and chopped
- ¼ cup cashews, raw, unsalted
- 1 cup chilled coconut milk, for serving
- 1 tablespoon chia seeds

Instructions:

1. Place all the ingredients through a blender.
2. Process well until smooth and creamy. If needed, add some water.
3. Serve and enjoy!

Recipe #4 High Energy Creamy Protein Smoothie

Citrus fruits are known for their high vitamin C and antioxidant properties, they are also great for boosting the immune system. They blend well with spinach and cashew milk to help you create a nutritious and delicious Vitamin C and iron packed recipe that also includes good fats and natural protein.

Servings: 2

Ingredients:

- 1 medium sized orange, peeled and chopped
- 1 medium sized grapefruit, peeled and chopped
- 1 cup baby spinach leaves
- 1 cup cashew milk

Instructions:

1. Place all the ingredients through a blender.
2. Process well until smooth and creamy. If needed, add some water.
3. Serve and enjoy!

Recipe #5 Apple Cinnamon Aphrodisiac Smoothie

Apples are very rich in essential antioxidants. They are also easily accessible and affordable. They blend well with arugula leaves while creating a tasty, balanced smoothie. Arugula is a natural aphrodisiac and so is the cinnamon. Chia seeds make this smoothie even more nutritious!

Servings: 2

Ingredients:

- 1 small red apple, chopped, seeds removed
- 1 small green apple, chopped, seeds removed
- A handful of fresh arugula leaves, washed
- 1 tablespoon chia seeds
- Half cup coconut milk

Instructions:

1. Place all the ingredients through a blender.
2. Process well until smooth and creamy. If needed, add some water. Serve and enjoy!

Recipe #6 Hydration Refreshment Protein Smoothie

The grapes are high in essential minerals and vitamin C and blend very well with arugula leaves. Perfect combo to enrich your diet with greens! Watermelon adds to natural sweetness and optimal hydration. Pistachios are high in protein, good fats and fiber.

Servings:2

Ingredients:

- Half cup grapes (red or white)
- Half cup arugula leaves
- Half cup watermelon chunks
- 4 tablespoons raw pistachio nuts
- 1 cup hazelnut milk or coconut milk

Instructions:

1. Place all the ingredients through a blender.
2. Process well until smooth and creamy.
3. If needed, add some water.
4. Serve and enjoy!

Recipe #7 Easy Sweet Green Smoothie

If you are having a hard time drinking green smoothies, this recipe will help fall in love with greens. This is a great breakfast option for sustained energy, and is very comforting because of its naturally sweet taste.

Servings: 2

Ingredients:

- 1 cup spinach leaves
- 1 small banana
- ¼ cup dates, pitted
- A handful of hazelnuts
- 1 cup hazelnut milk
- 1 tablespoon cinnamon powder

Instructions:

1. Place all the ingredients through a blender.
2. Process well until smooth and creamy. If needed, add some water.
3. Serve and enjoy!

Recipe #8 Sweet Anti-Inflammatory Smoothie

This recipe combines fresh cherries which are known for their high antioxidant properties with naturally sweet and highly alkalizing red bell peppers. Ginger adds to alkaline and anti-inflammatory properties that red bell pepper brings to the table.

Servings: 2

Ingredients:

- Half cup of fresh cherries, pitted
- 1 big red bell pepper, chopped, seeds removed
- 2-inch ginger, peeled
- 1 cup coconut water
- Half teaspoon maca powder
- 1 teaspoon chia seeds

Instructions:

1. Place all the ingredients through a blender.
2. Process well until smooth and creamy. If needed, add some water.
3. Serve and enjoy!

Recipe #9 Mediterranean Health Alkaline Smoothie

Tomatoes are high in vitamin C, antioxidants and essential minerals. Avocados are high in potassium and essential fats. Olives, nuts and herbs make this smoothie taste incredible while adding to its alkaline benefits.

Servings: 2

Ingredients:

- 1 cup cherry tomatoes
- 1 green bell pepper, chopped, seeds removed
- 1 ripe avocado, halved and pitted
- 1 tablespoon extra-virgin olive oil
- 1 garlic clove, peeled
- Half cup green olives, pitted
- 1 teaspoon fresh rosemary and thyme
- 1 tablespoon raw pistachio nuts
- Himalaya salt and black pepper to taste
- 2 cups water, filtered, preferably alkaline

Instructions:

1. Place all the ingredients through a blender.
2. Process well until smooth and creamy. If needed, add more water.

3. Serve and enjoy!

Suggestions:

This smoothie can be turned into a delicious soup. You can serve it raw, or lightly cooked.

The "smoothie soup" tastes really nice with some fresh olives, chopped onions and fresh parsley, chive or dill.

Yummy!

Enjoy!

Recipe #10 Cilantro Detox Smoothie

Cilantro is a great source of essential minerals and dietary fiber. The chia seeds add a healthy dose of fats and the cashew nuts provide the protein, as well as a little extra healthy fat.

Servings: 2

Ingredients:

- Half cup fresh cilantro leaves, well rinsed and dried off with kitchen towel
- 1 cucumber, peeled sliced
- A handful of raw cashew nuts
- 1 tablespoon chia seeds
- 1 cup of coconut milk
- Himalaya salt and black pepper to taste
- Half teaspoon turmeric powder

Instructions:

1. Place all the ingredients through a blender.
2. Process well until smooth and creamy. If needed, add some water.
3. Serve and enjoy!

Recipe #11 Pegan Weight Loss Smoothie

Himalaya salt makes this green smoothie taste delicious. You can also spice it up with some chili, curry, black pepper or cilantro!

This smoothie can be also served as a pegan smoothie soup, with some cashews or almonds.

Servings: 3-4

Ingredients:

- 2 cups coconut milk (unsweetened)
- 2 small avocados, peeled and pitted
- 1 big cucumber, peeled and chopped
- A handful of spinach
- Pinch of Himalaya salt to taste

Instructions:

1. Place all the ingredients in a blender.
2. Blend well.
3. Serve as a smoothie or a raw soup and enjoy!

Recipe #12 Keto Pegan Energy Detox Smoothie

This smoothie combines the best of keto, alkaline, vegan and paleo worlds! It tastes very refreshing and can also be served as a raw, healing soup.

Servings: 1-2

Ingredients:

- 1 cup thick coconut milk
- 1 avocado, peeled and pitted
- 1 small lime, peeled
- 2 tablespoons chia seeds or chia seed powder
- Half teaspoon curry powder
- Himalaya salt to taste (optional)
- 1 tablespoon coconut oil

Instructions:

1. Blend all the ingredients.
2. Pour your smoothie into a smoothie glass or a small soup bowl.
3. Sprinkle more curry powder or other spices on top.
4. Enjoy!

Recipe #13 Healthy Eyes Keto Pegan Smoothie

This creamy smoothie is a fantastic source of vitamin A to take care of your skin and eyes. Himalaya salt helps you add more alkaline minerals like Magnesium to your diet.

Servings: 2

Ingredients:

- 1 cup cashew milk, unsweetened, unsalted
- 2 tablespoons flax seed oil
- 1 cup fresh parsley leaves, washed
- 2 tablespoon fresh cilantro leaves, washed
- Black pepper (optional)
- Himalaya salt to taste
- 2 lime slices to garnish

Instructions:

1. Place all the ingredients in a blender.
2. Process until smooth.
3. Garnish with lime slices, serve and enjoy!

Recipe#14 Easy Lemon Detox Smoothie

This recipe provides a ton of Vitamin C and is very easy to make.

You can make it on the go, using a simple hand blender or a hand processor.

Servings: 2

Ingredients:

- 1 cup thick coconut milk (full fat)
- 1 tablespoon coconut oil
- 1 lemon, peeled and sliced
- 1 tablespoon chia seed powder
- 1 teaspoon cinnamon powder
- Optional – stevia to sweeten

Instructions:

1. Place all the ingredients in a blender.
2. Process until smooth.
3. Serve and enjoy!
4. If needed sweeten with stevia.

Recipe #15 Easy Vegan Paleo Relaxation Smoothie

I am a big fan of using herbal infusions in your smoothies. Herbal infusions are very inexpensive and can add more healing benefits to your vegan paleo smoothies. Chamomile is a great choice to help you relax on a deeper level!

Servings: 2

Ingredients:

- 1 cup chamomile tea (cooled down, use 1 teabag per cup)
- 1 small avocado, peeled and pitted
- 1 small lime, peeled and sliced
- Half cup almond milk
- 1 teaspoon cinnamon powder
- Stevia to sweeten if needed

Instructions:

1. Place all the ingredients in a blender.
2. Process until smooth.
3. Relax and enjoy!

Recipe #16 Spice It Up Mediterranean Smoothie

This smoothie is rich in good fats and protein and can be turned into a delicious, satisfying raw (or lightly cooked) soup. It's a great way to enrich your diet with green, alkaline veggies too!

Servings: 2

Ingredients:

- 2 green bell peppers, chopped, seeds removed
- Half avocado, peeled and pitted
- 1 small garlic clove, peeled
- Pinch of black pepper and chili
- 1 cup almond milk, unsweetened
- A handful of almonds, soaked in water for at least a few hours
- 1 tablespoon extra-virgin olive oil
- Himalaya salt to taste

Instructions:

1. Place all the ingredients in a blender.
2. Process until smooth, serve, and enjoy!

Recipe #17 Optimal Balance Smoothie

To make this smoothie, I recommend you use gloves.

Turmeric may make your hands and nails go orange and it's very hard to remove. You can also use turmeric powder or supplement instead.

Servings: 1-2

- 1 cup coconut milk, unsweetened
- 2-inch ginger, peeled
- 2-inch turmeric, peeled
- Half teaspoon Ashwagandha powder
- 1 banana, peeled
- Ice cubes and mint leaves to serve

Instructions:

1. Blend all the ingredients in a blender.
2. Serve with some ice cubes and fresh mint leaves.
3. Enjoy!

Recipe #18 Almond Protein Smoothie

This creamy smoothie combines plant-based protein with maca powder – a natural superfood with hormone-balancing properties.

Servings: 1-2

Ingredients:

- 1 cup coconut milk, unsweetened
- A handful of almonds (raw, unsweetened and soaked in filtered, alkaline water for a few hours)
- 1 green apple, chopped
- A handful of blueberries, fresh or frozen
- Half cup ice cubes
- Half teaspoon fresh maca powder

+ a few lime slices and ice cubes to serve if needed

Instructions:

1. Place all the ingredients in a blender.
2. Process until smooth.
3. Serve and enjoy!

Recipe #19 Creamy Energy Alkaline Pegan Smoothie

This creamy alkaline smoothie tastes delicious. It works really well if your goal is to restore energy and detoxify your body.

Servings: 2-3

Ingredients:

- 4 big cucumbers, peeled and roughly sliced
- Half cup radishes
- 1 cup of coconut milk
- 4 tablespoons cashews, chopped or powdered
- Pinch of Himalaya salt to taste
- Pinch of black pepper to taste

Instructions:

1. Place all the ingredients in a blender.
2. Process until smooth.
3. Pour into a smoothie glass or a small soup bowl.
4. Serve and enjoy!
5. Sprinkle the cashews and enjoy!

Recipe #20 Vegan Paleo Liver Lover Smoothie

Radishes are very alkalizing and good for your liver and immune system. They are also very refreshing! Perfect for a quick veggie smoothie (or a smoothie soup).

Servings: 1-2

Ingredients:

- 1 cup radishes, washed
- 1 cup full-fat coconut milk (no added sugar)
- 1 red bell pepper, chopped, seeds removed
- Pinch of Himalaya salt to taste
- Pinch of black pepper to taste
- Optional: red chili pepper

Instructions:

1. Blend all the ingredients.
2. Serve in a smoothie glass or in a soup bowl.

If you serve this smoothie as a soup, feel free to add in some nuts and seeds, for example pistachios. Yummy!

Recipe #21 Cilantro Antioxidant Smoothie

Cilantro is an amazing herb with potent antioxidant properties.

It blends really well with curry and greens. The result is a delicious, creamy, comforting smoothie!

Servings: 2-4

Ingredients:

- 1 cup coconut milk
- 1 cup cashew milk
- A handful of fresh cilantro leaves
- 2 red bell peppers, sliced and seeds removed
- 1 teaspoon curry powder
- Pinch of Himalaya salt to taste
- Pinch of black pepper powder to taste

Instructions:

1. Combine all the ingredients in a blender.
2. Process until smooth.
3. Add more salt or spices if needed.
4. Pour into a smoothie glass or a small soup bowl and enjoy!

Recipe #22 Vitamin C Sweetness Smoothie

This recipe creates the perfect balance by combining citric fruit with natural sweetness that dates and watermelon offer. I love this smoothie on a hot summer day.

Servings: 2

Ingredients:

- 1 big grapefruit, peeled and chopped
- 1 lime, peeled
- A handful of dates, pitted
- 1 cup fresh watermelon chunks
- 1 cup of coconut water
- A few mint leaves to garnish

Instructions:

1. Place all the ingredients in a blender.
2. Process until smooth.
3. Serve in a smoothie glass and garnish with a few mint leaves.
4. Drink to your health and enjoy!

Recipe #23 Superfood Protein Smoothie

This green protein smoothie is a fantastic way to help you feel energized! Spirulina is a natural source of protein and iron. A word of caution though- it may leave stains in your kitchen, so be careful while making this smoothie.

Servings: 2-3

Ingredients:

- Half cup kale leaves, washed
- 2 ripe pears, chopped
- 1 apple
- 1 inch of ginger, peeled
- Half teaspoon spirulina powder
- 1 tablespoon chia seeds
- 2 cups almond milk
- 2 slices of lime, to garnish
- Fresh ice cubes

Instructions:

1. Place all the ingredients (except lime) in a blender
2. Process until smooth.
3. Pour in a glass, add in some ice cubes.
4. Garnish with lime slices.

5. Serve and enjoy!

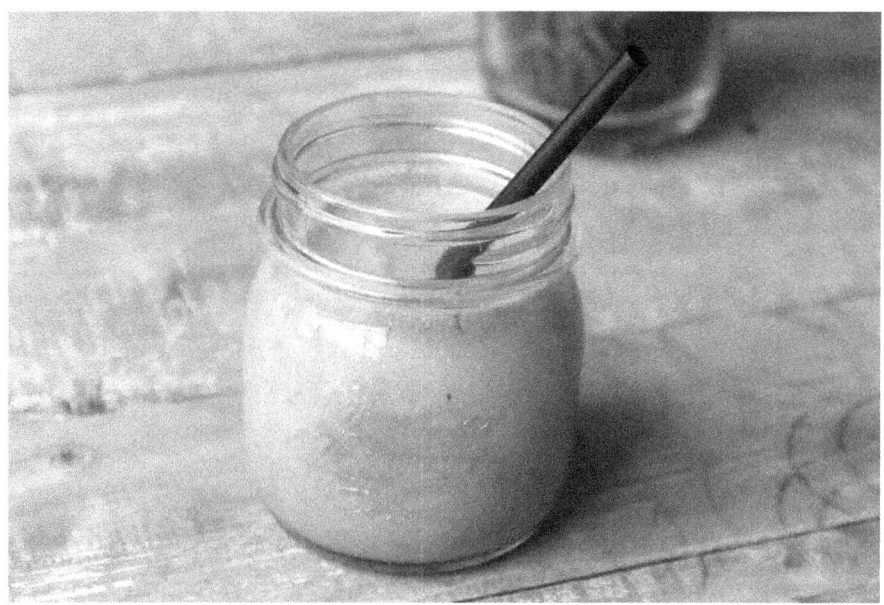

Recipe #24 Green Coconut Smoothie

This smoothie is a perfect nutritious, green pegan smoothie to enjoy first thing in the morning. Green tea can be added if you need a quick energy boost.

Servings: 2

Ingredients:

- 1 cup green tea, cooled down
- 2 green apples, peeled, and cut into smaller pieces
- 4 dates, pitted
- A handful of arugula leaves
- 1 teaspoon maca
- Optional – stevia to sweeten

Instructions:

1. Place all the ingredients in a blender.
2. Process until smooth.
3. If needed, add a bit more water.
4. Enjoy!

Recipe #25 Cinnamon Sweetness Smoothie

This smoothie is a great recipe to "recycle" some broccoli leftovers. I made this smoothie for a friend who couldn't even tell I used broccoli…

Servings: 2

Ingredients:

- A few broccoli florets, raw or steamed
- 3 oranges, peeled and cut into smaller pieces
- 1 cup almond milk
- 1 teaspoon cinnamon powder
- 1 tablespoon chia seeds

Instructions:

1. Blend all the ingredients.
2. If needed, add more water or vegan paleo milk.
3. Pour into a glass and enjoy!

Recipe #26 Green Tea Fat Burn Smoothie

This recipe offers a blend of highly alkalizing fruits and veggies combined with ginger to reduce inflammation.

Horsetail infusion is a natural remedy to ease water retention symptoms and feel lighter.

Servings: 2

Ingredients:

- 2 grapefruits, peeled and cut into smaller pieces
- 1-inch ginger, peeled
- 1 cup watermelon chunks
- 1 cup horsetail infusion, cooled down (use 1 teabag per cup)
- Ice cubes
- Mint leaves to garnish

Instructions:

1. Blend all the ingredients using a blender or a food processor.
2. Pour into a glass or a bowl.
3. Add in some mint leaves and ice cubes.
4. Enjoy!

Recipe #27 Natural Beauty Vegan Paleo Smoothie

This smoothie is an amazing, natural solution to help you have beautiful skin.

Servings: 2

Ingredients:

- 2 carrots, peeled and chopped
- 1 orange, peeled and cut into smaller pieces
- 1 lime, peeled and cut into smaller pieces
- 1 cup organic tomato juice
- 2-inch turmeric, peeled

Instructions:

1. Place all the ingredients through a blender.
2. Process well until smooth.
3. Enjoy!

Recipe #28 Spicy Antioxidant Smoothie

This smoothie is an amazing blend of alkaline raw foods, good fats and natural, vegan protein to help you stay energized, focused and full for hours!

Servings: 2

Ingredients:

- 6 tomatoes, peeled and cut into smaller pieces
- Handful of cilantro leaves
- 1 tablespoon chia seed powder
- 1-inch ginger, peeled
- Pinch of chili powder
- Himalaya salt to taste
- 1 cup water, filtered, preferably alkaline

Instructions:

1. Place all the ingredients through a blender.
2. Process well until smooth.
3. Enjoy!

Recipe #29 Hormone Rebalancer Smoothie

This smoothie recipe is a fantastic option if you don't like green smoothies, but you still want to experience all the health benefits of healthy, detox, vegan paleo blends.

Servings: 1-2

Ingredients:

- 1 big grapefruit, peeled and halved
- 1 green apple, peeled
- 1 kiwi, peeled
- 1 cup of coconut water
- 1 inch of ginger, peeled
- 1 tablespoon coconut oil
- Half teaspoon maca powder
- Stevia to sweeten, if desired

Instructions:

1. Blend all the ingredients in a blender.
2. Serve and enjoy!

Recipe #30 Mineral Dream Smoothie

This recipe can be used both as a smoothie as well as a soup.

It focuses on healthy, natural plant-based fats and hydrating veggies.

Servings: 1-2

Ingredients:

- 2 big cucumbers, peeled
- 1 small avocado, peeled and pitted
- A handful of parsley
- A handful of cilantro leaves, washed
- 1 cup of cashew milk, unsweetened, unsalted
- A handful of raw cashews
- Himalaya salt and black pepper to taste

Instructions:

1. Blend all the ingredients in a blender.
2. Serve in a smoothie glass or in a small soup bowl.
3. Enjoy!

Recipe #31 Creamy Alkaline Spicy Smoothie

This recipe also uses healing alkaline veggies like cauliflower, and, at the same time, adds in some garlic to help you strengthen your immune system. Cauliflower tastes amazing in smoothies; however, I recommend you cook it or steam it before blending it. What I really like about this recipe, is that its dense, creamy nature makes it very easy to turn it into a delicious soup.

Servings: 1-2

Ingredients:

- 1 cup cauliflower, cooked or steamed, cut into smaller pieces
- 1 cup thick coconut milk
- 1 tablespoon coconut oil
- Half avocado, peeled and pitted
- 2 garlic cloves, peeled and minced
- 1 red chili flake, or a pinch of chili powder
- Himalaya salt to taste
- Cilantro and parsley leaves to taste

Instructions:

1. Blend and enjoy!

Recipe #32 Fresh Basil Antioxidant Smoothie

The fresh basil is known for its anti-bacterial properties and has a unique flavor that pairs very well with the tomatoes and olives. This smoothie can also be turned into a soup.

Servings: 1-2

Ingredients:

- Half cup fresh basil leaves
- 1 cup fresh cherry tomatoes
- Half cup water, filtered, preferably alkaline
- Half cup black olives, pitted
- A handful of raw pine nuts
- Himalaya salt and black pepper to taste

Instructions:

1. Place all the ingredients in a blender.
2. Process until smooth.
3. If needed, add more water.
4. Serve as a smoothie or a soup.
5. Enjoy!

Recipe #33 Arugula Protein Smoothie

Arugula is high in alkaline minerals and dietary fiber; The Brazil nuts bring the protein, selenium and some essential fats to this party, while the avocado provides its potassium content and additional healthy fat. Oranges and watermelon add to natural sweetness and help neutralize the green taste of arugula (which I love anyway!).

Servings: 2

Ingredients:

- 1 cup of fresh arugula leaves
- A handful of raw brazil nuts, roughly chopped
- Half of a ripe avocado, sliced
- 2 oranges
- Half cup watermelon chunks
- 1 cup water (filtered, preferably alkaline) or coconut water
- Mint leaves to garnish

Instructions:

1. Blend all the ingredients until smooth.
2. Pour into a big smoothie glass and garnish with fresh mint leaves.
3. Serve and enjoy!

Recipe #34 Carrot Orange Protein Pegan Smoothie

Carrots are high in beta carotene and vitamin A; they contain essential antioxidants and are also a great source of dietary fiber. Oranges boost this smoothie with Vitamin C, dates add to natural sweetness. Almonds and chia add good protein and fats. This smoothie will keep you going for many hours!

Servings: 2

Ingredients:

- 2 big carrots, peeled
- 1 big orange, peeled and cut into smaller pieces
- Handful of dates, chopped
- Handful of raw almonds, roughly chopped
- 2 tablespoons chia seeds
- 1 cup coconut milk

Instructions:

1. Place all the ingredients in a blender.
2. Process until smooth.
3. If needed, add more water.
4. Enjoy!

Recipe #35 Easy Refreshment Smoothie

Cucumber has a high liquid content so it's great for helping maintain hydration throughout the afternoon; it is also known to be a great addition to a diet that's keeping a healthy, glowing skin in mind. It blends well with apples and watermelon. Cinnamon makes it smoothie naturally sweet and maca is a natural stimulant and hormone balancer.

Servings: 2

Ingredients

- 1 small red apple, cored and sliced
- 1 small green apple, cored and sliced
- 1 big cucumber, peeled and sliced
- 1 cup watermelon chunks
- 1 cup ice cubes
- 1 teaspoon maca powder
- 1 teaspoon cinnamon powder

Instructions:

1. Blend all the ingredients.
2. Serve and enjoy!

Recipe #36 Delicious Green Mediterranean Smoothie

Zucchini is a great source of dietary fiber and essential minerals and is one of those vegetables that can be enjoyed both raw and cooked. It blends well with all kinds of herbs and veggies. This smoothie is super easy to make and offers a great option if you want to make a green smoothie that is a bit different.

Servings: 2

Ingredients:

- 2 zucchinis, peeled (raw or cooked)
- Half cup raw cherry tomatoes
- Half cup green olives, pitted
- 1 tablespoon extra-virgin olive oil
- 1 tablespoon raw seed mix
- Optional: Himalaya salt and black pepper to taste
- 1 cup water, filtered, preferably alkaline
- 1 cup organic tomato juice or carrot juice

Instructions:

1. Blend all the ingredients.
2. Serve and enjoy!

Recipe #37 Super Irion Smoothie

The combination of spinach and sweet peppers in this smoothie is another example of how the body's ability to absorb the high iron content of the spinach is boosted by pairing it with another vegetable that is high in vitamin C. This smoothie can also be enjoyed as a nice, raw, or warm healing soup.

Servings: 2

Ingredients:

- 1 cup fresh baby spinach leaves
- 1 red bell pepper, sliced
- A handful of raw pistachios, roughly chopped
- Half of a ripe avocado
- 1 cup coconut or nut milk of your choice
- Half cup of water, filtered, preferably alkaline
- Himalaya salt to taste (optional)

Instructions:

1. Place all the ingredients in a blender.
2. Process until smooth.
3. If needed, add more water.
4. Enjoy!

Recipe #38 Good Fat Good Protein Pegan Smoothie

Many people are too scared to give the pegan diet a try because they think they will miss protein and fats.

Well...the pegan diet is not just about the fruits and vegetables. This smoothie is the best proof.

Servings: 2

Ingredients:

- 1 ripe avocado, halved and pitted
- 1 tablespoon mixed micro herbs
- A handful of raw pine nuts
- A handful of almonds, soaked
- A handful of dates, pitted
- 1 tablespoon raw seed mix
- 1 cup coconut milk or nut milk

Instructions:

1. Place all the ingredients in a blender.
2. Process until smooth.
3. Enjoy!

Recipe #39 Creamy Papaya Refreshment Smoothie

Papaya has a light, sweet taste and is great for digestion. The cashew nuts add a nice crunch and a hearty dose of protein. This smoothie tastes delicious chilled, and offers an amazing refreshment on a hot, summer day.

Servings: 2

Ingredients:

- 1 cup diced fresh papaya
- Half cup raw cashew nuts, roughly chopped
- 1 tablespoon coconut shavings
- 1 cup cashew milk (you can also use filtered water or coconut water)
- 1 cup ice cubes

Instructions:

1. Place all the ingredients in a blender.
2. Process until smooth.
3. Serve chilled.
4. Enjoy!

Recipe #40 Easy Fat Burn Pineapple Smoothie

The pineapple goes very well with the green tea and grapefruit. All these ingredients combine some really powerful fat-burning properties and make it a perfect detox smoothie to help you look and feel amazing.

Servings: 2

Ingredients:

- 1 cup fresh pineapple, diced
- 1 grapefruit, peeled and chopped
- 1-inch ginger, peeled
- 1 cup green tea, cooled down (use 1 teabag per cup)
- Optional: stevia to sweeten

Instructions:

1. Place all the ingredients in a blender.
2. Process until smooth.
3. If needed, sweeten with stevia.
4. Enjoy!

Recipe #41 Natural Detox Carrot Soup Style Smoothie

With this amazing smoothie recipe, you can boost your immune system with massive amounts of vitamins C and A. Ginger is great for digestive problems and acts as a natural anti-inflammatory. You can also enjoy this smoothie as a delicious, raw, healing soup.

Serves: 4

Ingredients:

- 4 large carrots, peeled and chopped
- Fresh juice of 1 orange
- Fresh juice of 1 lime
- 1 mango, peeled, pitted and chopped
- 2 inches of ginger
- 1 big onion
- 1 red bell pepper
- 2 garlic cloves
- Half cup cilantro, chopped
- 2 cups coconut milk
- 1 tablespoon avocado oil
- Half cup sunflower seeds
- Himalayan/sea salt to taste

Instructions:

1. Place all the ingredients (except cilantro, sunflower seeds and oil) in a blender. Blend until smooth and creamy.
2. Add a pinch of Himalayan salt to taste. Sprinkle some avocado oil, cilantro and sunflower seeds over the soup.
3. Enjoy!

Recipe #42 Exotic Soup Style Smoothie

Greens are super alkalizing so use them in your pegan smoothies. You can use your blender to create nutrient-packed, dense smoothies almost like soups or vegetable creams. They are quick and easy to prepare and a fantastic way of eating in the summer. In the winter, you may heat them up slightly, it's up to you!

Serves: 2

Ingredients:

- 1 cup coconut or any nut milk of your choice
- 1 cup water, filtered
- A handful of cilantro leaves
- Half cup arugula leaves
- 1 cucumber, peeled
- 1 big garlic clove
- Half cup of radish
- 2 big tomatoes
- A handful of cashews (soaked in water for a few hours)
- 1/2 tsp. turmeric powder
- 1/4 tsp black pepper (real game changer as it helps your body get all the anti-inflammatory benefits that turmeric powder offers)
- A pinch of Himalayan salt
- 1 tablespoon coconut oil

- 1 tablespoon fresh lime juice
- 1 tablespoon lemon juice

Instructions:

1. Blend well.
2. Squeeze some fresh lime or lemon juice into the mixture, and enjoy!
3. Serve as a smoothie or a soup.

Recipe #43 Dried Fruit Dream Smoothie

Easy, sweet and delicious!

Servings: 2

Ingredients:

- 4 carrots, peeled
- ¼ cup of dried fruit of your choice (unsweetened)
- 1 cup coconut milk or nut milk
- 1 tablespoon apple cider vinegar or lemon juice
- 1 teaspoon cinnamon powder
- Half teaspoon maca powder

Instructions:

1. Blend and enjoy.
2. This smoothie makes an excellent dessert recipe.

Recipe #44 White Chia Smoothie

This delicious white-creamy style smoothie combines sweet bananas and not so sweet lemons to create an amazing, balanced taste.

It also contains chia seeds and a myriad of other superfoods to help you look and feel amazing!

Serves: 1-2

Ingredients:

- 2 small bananas, peeled
- 2 small lemons, peeled
- 1 small pear
- A few dates, pitted
- 2 tablespoons chia seeds
- 1 cup coconut milk
- Half cup water, filtered, preferably alkaline
- 1 tablespoon coconut oil
- Half teaspoon maca powder
- Half teaspoon Ashwagandha powder
- 2 tablespoons almond powder

Instructions:

1. Blend all the ingredients.
2. Serve and enjoy!

Recipe #45 Delicious Thai Style Smoothie

This recipe is one of my favorite oriental smoothies.

Perfect if you want to try something different!

Serves: 2

Ingredients:

- 2 medium zucchinis, peeled and chopped
- 2 carrots, peeled and chopped
- 1 green onion, peeled and chopped
- 1 green bell pepper, chopped
- 1 cup red cabbage, chopped
- 1 cup thick coconut milk
- 1 cup coconut water
- A handful of cashews, raw
- 1 lime, peeled
- 1 teaspoon Ashwagandha powder (optional)
- A pinch of chili powder
- A pinch of black pepper
- A pinch of Himalayan salt
- A few dates, pitted

Instructions:

1. Place ingredients in a blender and process until smooth.
2. If too thick, add a little water.
3. Serve as a smoothie, soup, dip or sauce.
4. Enjoy!

Recipe #46 Nutritious Vanilla Smoothie

This smoothie combines optimal nutrition with delicious taste!

Serves 1-2

Ingredients:

- 1 natural vanilla bean
- 1 cup of raw cashew milk
- 1 small banana, peeled
- 2 tablespoons nutritional yeast
- 1 lime, peeled
- 1 pear, chopped
- 1 apple, chopped
- A handful of raw cashews
- 1 teaspoon coconut oil

Instructions:

1. Take the vanilla bean and press it flat with your fingers.
2. Then take a knife and gently split the vanilla bean open and scoop out the fresh vanilla specs with a spoon.
3. Pour the cashew milk into the blender.
4. Add the banana into the blender.
5. Then put the vanilla and the nutritional yeast in the mix.
6. Add the apple and pear.

7. Then add the coconut oil and cashews.
8. Blend the mix well so everything is pureed. When smoothie is at desired flavor, pour the smoothie into a glass and serve chilled.
9. Enjoy!

Recipe #47 Seduction Cinnamon Smoothie

This smoothie combines the sweetness of cinnamon with apples. To make this recipe, you can use raw apples (quick version), or cooked apples (you can cook them in coconut oil and then blend them). The second option is great if you crave some comfort food!

The pegan diet also incorporates cooked food. The basic rule is always listen to your body, it knows.

Servings: 1-2

Ingredients:

- 2 teaspoons of cinnamon powder
- 1 cup coconut milk
- 2 big red apples, chopped
- 4 dates, pitted
- Optional: a teaspoon of green powders of your choice.

Instructions:

1. Blend and enjoy!
2. This smoothie is just perfect if you are craving something sweet.

Recipe #48 Ashwagandha Herbal Delight Smoothie

This smoothie uses fennel infusion for optimal taste and benefits. Fennel is helpful in natural weight loss, relaxation and it also helps strengthen your immune system.

Servings: 1-2

Ingredients:

- 1 cup fennel tea, cooled down (use one teabag per cup)
- 1 cup coconut milk
- 1 frozen banana, peeled
- 1 apple, chopped
- 4 dates, pitted
- Half cup of blueberries
- 2 tablespoons lime juice
- 1 teaspoon moringa powder

Instructions:

1. Place all the ingredients in a blender.
2. Process until smooth.
3. Serve chilled.
4. Enjoy!

Conclusion

Sign up for my vegan recipe email newsletter to receive this free complimentary smoothie guide:

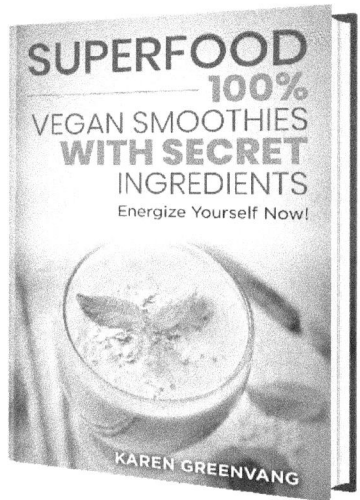

Sign up for this free guide and email updates below:

www.yourwellnessbooks.com/karen-smoothies

(I hate spam and annoying marketing emails as much as you do and I honor your privacy, I promise to send out 100% love & positivity-based emails).

Problems with your sign up and free gift?

Please email me: karenveganbooks@gmail.com

Conclusion

Thank you for reading this recipe booklet to the end.

I hope that with so many pegan smoothie recipes you will feel inspired to take positive action on your vegan wellness journey.

The beauty of incorporating nutritious pegan foods into your daily diet is that you are making simple, yet sustainable changes that will work for your health and wellbeing, long-term.

If you enjoyed my book, it would be greatly appreciated if you left an honest review on the Amazon platform so that others can receive the same benefits you have.

Your review can help other people take this important step to take care of their health and inspire them to start a new chapter in their lives.

I'd be thrilled to hear from you. I would love to know your favorite recipe(s).

Conclusion

➔ Questions about this book? Email me at:

  karenveganbooks@gmail.com

Thank You for your time,

Love & Light,

Until next time-

Karen Vegan Greenvang

Conclusion

Special Offer from Karen- VIP Reader Newsletter

Are you looking for more vegan health inspiration?

Join my free email newsletter today and start receiving my best vegan tips, recipes and resources:

Visit:

www.YourWellnessBooks.com/karen

to sign up now.

(As my VIP reader, you will be the first one to learn about my new books at super discounted prices + giveaways +discounts).

Join now, it's free:

www.YourWellnessBooks.com/karen

I am looking forward to connecting with you helping you on your journey.

Conclusion

More Books by Karen Greenvang

Pegan Diet Cookbook

Alkaline Vegan Drinks

Vegan Baking

Spiralizer Cookbook

Vegan Protein Smoothies & Green Smoothies

And many more books and eBooks available at:

www.amazon.com/author/karengreenvang

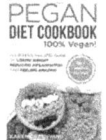 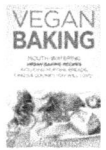 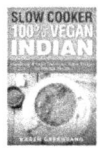 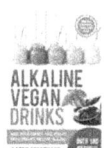 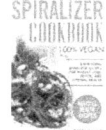

Conclusion

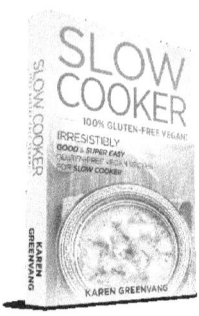

Karen's personal email is:

karenveganbooks@gmail.com

Always happy to connect with you,

With love and light,

Karen

www.ingramcontent.com/pod-product-compliance
Lightning Source LLC
Chambersburg PA
CBHW071753080526
44588CB00013B/2225